# THE FOETAL CIRCULATION

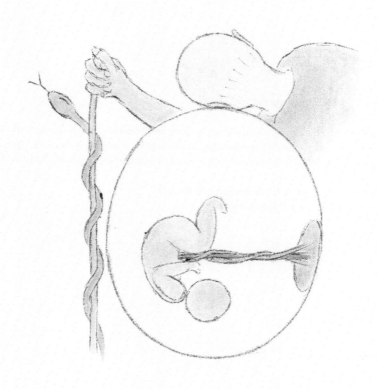

*6ᵗʰ and final edition*

*Alan Gilchrist*

AuthorHouse™ UK
1663 Liberty Drive
Bloomington, IN 47403  USA
www.authorhouse.co.uk
UK TFN: 0800 0148641 (Toll Free inside the UK)
UK Local: 02036 956322 (+44 20 3695 6322 from outside the UK)

Because of the dynamic nature of the Internet, any web addresses or links contained in this book may have changed since publication and may no longer be valid. The views expressed in this work are solely those of the author and do not necessarily reflect the views of the publisher, and the publisher hereby disclaims any responsibility for them.

Any people depicted in stock imagery provided by Getty Images are models, and such images are being used for illustrative purposes only.
Certain stock imagery © Getty Images.

This book is printed on acid-free paper.

ISBN: 978-1-6655-8143-1 (sc)
ISBN: 978-1-6655-8142-4 (e)

Print information available on the last page.

Published by AuthorHouse 03/27/2021

authorHOUSE®

This little book is dedicated to my parents, James and Ivy Gilchrist, and to my wife Pauline.

# Acknowledgements

The 5th edition of this book was produced in cramped quarters when I was living with my son Andrew and his wife Kim and their three sons. Since October 2018 I have been living by myself in a little flat which has given me more space to live and work in. Andrew has been a great help in the transition and keeps an eye on me from time to time, while I miss Kim's expertise assistance on my computer. Most important was having the space to fit in a deep freezer in which I could store my animal dissections, instead of just bottling them in formalin and keeping them in the garden. The move seems to have helped me to think more clearly and this final edition introduces many new ideas. In the 5th edition I told you about my back injury which prevented me from working on one of the lambs, but though I am less mobile now I have been able to examine more foetal lambs and complete this edition. I now have a little scooter which is a great boon; I can whizz round to the shops at 3.8 mph and get all I need without waiting for buses. I have tried to improve the quality of my diagrams, but some of the letters of the captions are still wobbly.

I am very grateful to Sophia Anderton, Head of Publishing & Digital Learning in the British Institute of Radiology, who has very kindly permitted me to publish details of two articles from the British Journal of Radiology. To Oswestry farmer Graham Jones, I again give many thanks for providing me with stillborn lambs which have played a large part in helping to unravel the hidden mysteries of the foetal circulation. In this regard I must also thank Kevin Battams of Battams Butchery in Oswestry for providing me with parts of the postnatal lamb. I still run into difficulties with my laptop, but I have been helped at home by Ben Hillidge of the Reliant Company in Oswestry. Nigel of Cartridge World Oswestry has again come to my rescue and solved my printer problems. A special mention and thanks for John Quinn, photographer in Oswestry for the high quality of his work in reproducing my diagrams in high resolution. This little book conceived in Africa and nurtured in England, has been safely delivered after a long and difficult labour, in Oswestry. It is a newly born offspring of Oswestry, which is now able to receive visitors. I invite you to come and see it. Alan.

# References

The Foetal Circulation. The Personal Account by a Zimbabwe Family Practitioner. By Alan Gilchrist. Printed in Zimbabwe by Graphtec Zimbabwe.2011.

A Visit to Nyasaland/The Foetal Circulation. By Alan Gilchrist. Printed by YOUCAXTON PUBLICATIONS. 2014.

The Foetal Circulation Reflections. By Alan Gilchrist. Printed by YOUCAXTON PUBLICATIONS. 2015.

The Foetal Circulation. By Alan Gilchrist. Published by AUTHORHOUSE. 2017.

The foetal Circulation. 5th Edition. By Alan Gilchrist. Published by AUTHORHOUSE. 2018.

Foetal and Neonatal Physiology. By G. S. DAWES. Published by YEAR BOOK MEDICAL PUBLISHERS, INC. Chicago. 1968.

Textbook of Medical Physiology by Guyton and Hall Twelfth Edition. The Heart Sounds.

An Apology.

I was sorry to see on page 25 of the 6th edition that a picture of a lamb's heart had obscured part of the text. I had missed this error when I was reading the proof copy. Fortunately, only a few copies were distributed, and printing has now resumed without the error. The interruption has given me the opportunity to make several changes, and especially important is my embellishment of the birth changes.

John Quinn, a dedicated fellow professional, has come out of retirement to help me sort out a few things, which include: kindly advice, reproducing the diagrams in high definition, replacing the diagrams and pictures and ensuring for the book a safe passage to the publisher in a presentable condition. Alan.

# Contents

Part One.
The Plan.    P. 1

Part Two.
The Sections.    P. 16

The Circulation for the Placenta.    P. 16
The Venturi/ Segregation.    P. 17
The Circulation for the Upper Body.    P. 18
The Circulation for the Lower Body.    P. 18
The Junction.    P. 19
The Foramen Ovale.    P. 20
The Left Atrium.    P. 25
The Postnatal Right Atrium.    P. 26
The Lungs.    P. 26
The Liver.    P. 27
The Block.    P. 27

Part Three.
The Foetal Heart Sounds.    P. 28

Part Four.
The Birth Changes.    P. 29

The Foetal Circulation.

Part One.

## The Plan.

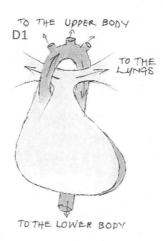

In the postnatal creature, which I call a postnate, Diagram 1, D 1. the two great arteries which leave the heart together curve upwards; the pulmonary trunk from the right ventricle ending abruptly by bifurcating into the two pulmonary arteries for the lungs, while the aorta from the left ventricle supplies the upper body and curves over the pulmonary arteries to pass down behind them as the descending aorta to supply the lower body. The blood in the postnate is either venous or arterial: venous before it reaches the lungs and arterial afterwards.

In the foetus, D 2, the arrangement is different. The pulmonary trunk extends beyond the pulmonary arteries, giving a little for the unexpanded lungs, and ends by joining the aorta. The blood in the descending aorta which supplies the lower body and the placenta is therefore a mixture of venous and arterial.

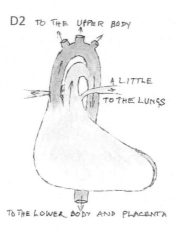

The re-oxygenated arterial-type blood returning from the placenta in the umbilical vein, reaches the liver and enters the upper part of the inferior vena cava, which carries it to the heart. D 3.

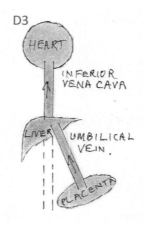

According to the orthodox accounts of the foetal circulation, this upper part of the inferior vena cava also carries the venous return from the lower body of the foetus, separated by streaming from the blood from the placenta, and both streams enter the right atrium. The arterial stream is then said to pass through the foramen ovale into the left atrium. D 4.

There is no doubt that some streaming of the blood does occur in blood vessels, but not of the respiratory gases in solution. Where there are different levels or pressures of oxygen and carbon-dioxide in solution close together, there is a rapid movement of each gas

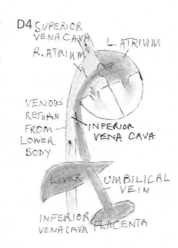

from higher to lower, resulting in equilibrium and a homogeneous mixture of both, with pressures midway between the two extremes. It is this extremely fast reaction which allows us to carry out the most strenuous of activities in the best of health. There was a very good demonstration of it during the Oxford and Cambridge boat races on 7th April 2019. Some of the crews had sensors on their big toes which recorded their heart rates going up to more than 200 beats per minute. Their respiratory rates were also high, probably approaching the stroke rates of the oars at 40 breaths per minute. The flow of air in the lung airways, and the flow of blood in the capillaries of the lung respiratory zone would pass each other at excessive speeds, and in the briefest moment of time carbon-dioxide would pass from the lungs to the air, and oxygen would pass from the air into the blood. Otherwise the crews would succumb from oxygen lack and excess carbon-dioxide. And if two separate streams of arterial and venous blood were to enter the foetal inferior vena cava side by side, the same reaction would lead immediately to a mixed homogeneous stream with a low oxygen level and excess carbon-dioxide which would kill the foetus. *Separation of the respiratory gases by streaming cannot occur; it is a myth.*

D 5 Shows the fast reaction in the lungs. D 6 shows how two streams side by side quickly become homogeneous.

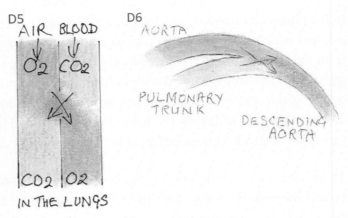

We can therefore rule out any possibility of a venous stream joining the arterial placental stream if the foetus is to remain healthy and there can be only one stream, the placental. We can also be certain that the placental stream would lead to the left atrium; any suggestion of it leading to the right atrium would be absurd. D 7.

It is the venous return from the lower body which would lead to the right atrium, but not together with the placental stream. The inferior vena cava must be separated functionally in the region of the liver into two parts: the upper to supply the left atrium with arterial blood and the lower to supply the right atrium with venous blood, and the lower return must reach the right atrium by an alternative route.

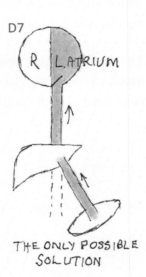

After the placental stream has passed through the left side of the heart it joins the venous flow from the right heart *beyond* the heart, *not proximally,* as I have shown you in diagram 2, and the mixed stream must contain the venous return from both parts of the foetus because all the venous return must be replenished by the placenta. We therefore know that the lower venous return would have already entered the right atrium by an alternative route and joined the upper return. We also know that the mixed blood in the descending aorta would be homogeneous. D 6.

I am surprised by how many men of science have accepted the concept of separation by streaming. If it were true, which it is not of course, it would have been a hit and miss affair which would not have lasted five minutes. It seems to me, from what I know of heredity and the replication of the double helix, that when we were first planted on this earth long, long ago, we were meant to last. Homo sapiens then, homo sapiens now and homo sapiens for as long as we remain here.

Recently I have been able to obtain from the British Institute of Radiology a copy of an article published in the British Journal of Radiology in 1939. Vol. XII, No. 141. It demonstrated with intravascular injections of radio-opaque substances and radiological cinematography, the circulation of the blood in live foetal lambs. It reveals the difficult complicated pioneering work performed by A. E. Barclay, Sir Joseph Barcroft,

D. H. Barron and K. J. Franklin, in the Nuffield Institute for Medical Research, Oxford, and shows for the first time, the circulation not only in live foetal lambs with x-rays, but probably in the unborn child without exposure to radiation.

Their work would have been carried out just before the outbreak of the second world war, and we must realise that at that time there was a strict anti-abortion law, with few human foetuses available for research. Only a year before, an eminent obstetrician had been arrested by the police for terminating the three month's pregnancy in a fourteen-year old girl who had been raped by five British soldiers. The Oxford work would have been a landmark in the investigation of the foetus, and the results would have been accepted as the norm. The quality of the work was of the highest calibre, and the photographs they have allowed us to see are very valuable, but the conclusions reached were mainly wrong.

Many of the pictures show radio-opaque material flowing down the superior vena cava to the right atrium. But there is one which shows the same sort of material flowing up the inferior vena cava. The article says: 'In the foetus, the inferior caval flow is composed of oxygenated blood returning to the heart from the placenta *via* the umbilical vein, and venous blood from the lower segment.' This is an assumption; they could only be certain that the blood flowing up the inferior vena cava contained the oxygenated blood from the placenta. It then says: 'We have not as yet traced the course taken by this venous blood, our experiments having been confined to the demonstration of the flow from the umbilical vein.' It continues: 'The main portion of this stream, after entering the right auricle, passes through the foramen ovale to the left auricle and left ventricle.' (The word 'auricle' is now no longer used and has been substituted by 'atrium'). This is another assumption. It is quite impossible to make out the details of the atria, and in any case the picture they show is different from the others which do show the right atrium, and therefore the mainstream may have entered the left atrium, not the right.

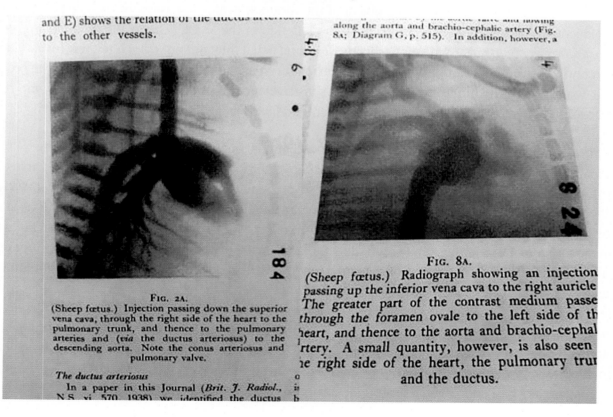

and E) shows the relation of the ductus arteriosus to the other vessels.

FIG. 2A.
(Sheep fœtus.) Injection passing down the superior vena cava, through the right side of the heart to the pulmonary trunk, and thence to the pulmonary arteries and (*via* the ductus arteriosus) to the descending aorta. Note the conus arteriosus and pulmonary valve.

*The ductus arteriosus*
In a paper in this Journal (*Brit. J. Radiol.*, N.S. vi. 570, 1938) we identified the ductus

along the aorta and brachio-cephalic artery (Fig. 8A; Diagram G, p. 515). In addition, however, a

FIG. 8A.
(Sheep fœtus.) Radiograph showing an injection passing up the inferior vena cava to the right auricle. The greater part of the contrast medium passes through the foramen ovale to the left side of the heart, and thence to the aorta and brachio-cephalic artery. A small quantity, however, is also seen in the right side of the heart, the pulmonary trunk and the ductus.

I am grateful to the authors for having shown the results of their work; the pictures are quite extraordinary and allow me to draw my own conclusions, which differ from theirs. I have introduced two of their photographs here. The first shows the opaque material flowing down the superior vena cava to the right atrium, while the second shows the injection flowing up the inferior vena cava. They say this flow in the inferior vena cava goes to the right auricle, but as I have said earlier, it can only go to the left atrium. Further on they say: 'In addition, however, a certain quantity is detached from the main stream in the right auricle and is carried through the right atrio-ventricular (tricuspid) valve to the right ventricle and pulmonary trunk.' There is no mention of streaming here, but is it not inferred? Earlier in the article the authors point out that none of the blood from the superior vena cava which enters the right atrium passes through the foramen ovale, but the blood which enters the right atrium from the inferior vena cava does pass through the foramen ovale. This suggests to me that these two 'right' atria are two different atria, and that the blood from the inferior vena cava may not have entered the right atrium, but the left.

If we consider the four streams of blood flowing to the left atrium from the lungs in the postnate as one single stream, then there are three streams leading to the heart and two atria to receive them. Both venae cavae lead venous blood to the right atrium, and the lungs lead arterial blood to the left atrium. You will see later that in the foetus the arrangement is fundamentally the same, with the arterial stream for the left atrium coming from the placenta instead of the lungs. But the authors here are in effect saying that all three streams lead to the right atrium, with no stream leading directly to the left. This is preposterous. It probably led to the false concept of right heart dominance, for which there was no evidence.

Although this article revealed parts of the foetal circulation which confirmed what was known, it failed to identify the unknown vitally important features which are necessary to understand it all. It seems to me that the authors were more intent on confirming the old wrong orthodox ideas rather than challenging them. At the beginning they say: 'the object of the foramen ovale is to allow re-oxygenated blood from the placenta to pass from the right auricle to the left side of the heart.' *This is the fundamental error of the orthodox accounts,* as I will show shortly. It is a pity that they did not complete their investigation of the venous flow in the lower segment of the inferior vena cava; it may have solved many of the problems. Their work was of the highest quality, but not sensitive enough to discriminate between some parts of the heart chambers and the vessels and has several misleading assumptions.

In 1968 G. S. Dawes produced a book called 'Foetal and Neonatal Physiology', published by Year Book Medical Publishers, INC. Chicago, which held the copyright. With some difficulty I have been able to get a copy. It appears that Geoffrey Dawes would have devoted much of his professional life to the investigation of the foetus, and the book covers it in depth from many angles. The results of his work were based on his investigations, also carried out in the Nuffield Institute for Medical Research in Oxford, and he used the same technique of cineangiography on live foetal lambs used by the previous Oxford group. I have been unable to trace the present owners of the copyright of this book, if there are any, so I am not allowed to discuss in detail its contents. However, I can say that as regards the plan of the circulation, his work was inferior to the earlier Oxford work because he does not show us his photographs, *only diagrams of his conclusions,* which are quite bizarre and awfully wrong. Some are more complicated than the Hampton Court Maze, which would make it impossible for the foetus to change quickly into a neonate at the moment of birth. He appears to have laboured all along under the fundamental misconceptions of the plan, as his predecessors had done, which is a pity, because his ideas are still quoted as the orthodox in standard medical publications. I am able to condemn with confidence the conclusions of both Oxford researches, because of some of my own investigations carried out in Africa some fifty or so years ago, supported by animal dissections performed more recently in England.

Since my student days I had been concerned how two streams of blood: one arterial and the other venous, could enter the same chamber of the heart and remain separate. Then in 1965 when I was working in the Fort Victoria hospital in Rhodesia, I was given the answer. (In 1980 Rhodesia became the independent country of Zimbabwe, and Fort Victoria was re-named Mazvingo). For three out of the four years spent there I was single-handed. Then, as well as caring for the hospital patients, I became involved with a huge amount of forensic work for the police. Every few days, or even daily, a police Land Rover with an aluminium coffin on its roof would drive up with a body for me to examine. I sometimes spent more time in the mortuary than in the wards. The clinical work on the one hand and the forensic cases on the other combined to make the whole a unique medical experience without equal: four years of forensic medicine side by side with four years of clinical medicine of great diversity. I have not told you these things only to show you some of the interesting happenings of that time, though they are interesting; I was now doing the work of a forensic pathologist, and it was the work in the mortuary which led to my solving the riddle of the two streams in the right atrium.

In April 1965 a baby girl was delivered in the hospital under my care and died because we were unable to make her breathe. Her body had been taken to the hospital mortuary, where not surprisingly I was performing a police post-mortem. I was engrossed in my work, but my thoughts gradually turned to her. If she had not breathed, would she have been like a foetus which does not breathe in utero, and would her circulation still be in the foetal condition? I finished the post-mortem, went over to her and opened her chest. The heart lay horizontally above the raised diaphragm with the unexpanded lungs on each side. It is a very strange thing; none of the accounts I have read mentions the raised diaphragm and the position of the thoracic organs. I assume it is the normal arrangement contributing to the economy of space, so important in the little curled up intrauterine creature. D 8.

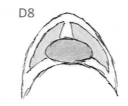
D8

I removed the heart and lungs together, put them in preserving fluid, took them home and later examined them. Straight away I could see how the streams were separated. It was an emotional moment for me; the first time I had examined a foetal heart which gave me the answer I was seeking. Why had it not been revealed before? I cast my eyes upwards. Had I been guided? The oval mouth of the inferior vena did lead to the right atrium, but not into it. Instead it was closely and accurately applied round the foramen ovale in the atrial septum and led into the left atrium, not the right, and in life the placental flow would have entered the left atrium without having entered the right atrium at all. D 9. The wall of the right atrium was folded inwards, making a tube which ran above the inferior vena cava from the superior vena cava to the right ventricle, and in life the venous return in the right atrium would have flowed above the placental stream below. D 10.

The streams are therefore separated because only one of them, the venous stream from the superior vena cava, enters the right atrium. The arterial placental stream in the inferior vena cava leads into the left atrium below the other, ensuring that inter-atrial flow does not occur. *Now we see the fundamental error in the orthodox accounts: whether it be from the lungs of the baby or the placenta of the foetus, the oxygen from the respiratory organ goes directly to the left atrium. It is a principle.*

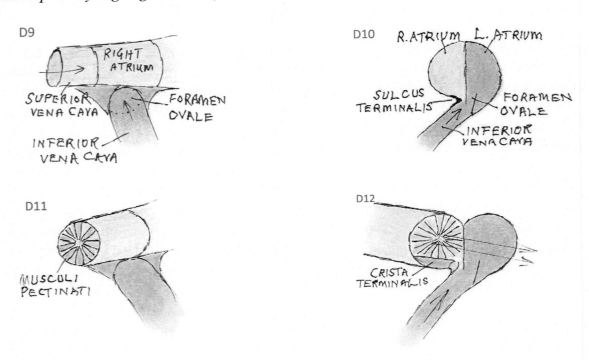

There was a groove between the tubular right atrium and the inferior vena cava which was the sulcus terminalis. When I looked at the upper end of the tube, I could see muscular flaps arranged radially inside it. I opened the tube: the flaps were the musculi pectinati. D 11.

There was a thickened bar of tissue running down the tube opposite the sulcus terminalis, which was the crista terminalis. It ran along the top of the inferior vena cava giving support to that vessel in its contact with the atrial septum. I imagined the cardiac impulse from the pacemaker near the upper end of the crista spreading down the tube, causing the flaps to contract rhythmically in waves and milking the blood down to the right ventricle above the placental stream below. D 12.

I made careful drawings of the specimen then showed it to Pauline and explained how the two streams were separated. She said: "It's like a flyover." Now I hadn't thought of that. What an apt description. D's 9—12.

After leaving the flyover the two streams enter their respective ventricles and the arterial is pumped into the aorta, while the venous enters the pulmonary trunk, the end of which is known as the ductus arteriosus. They then meet at the aorto-ductal junction, which I call 'the junction'. Now, I had been concerned about the way the ductus is shown in various articles to enter the aorta. I had imagined it to be a sort of 'T' junction, and after solving the riddle of the two streams I paid special attention to the junction and found that the ductus did not enter the aorta; there was no 'T' junction. That is only a

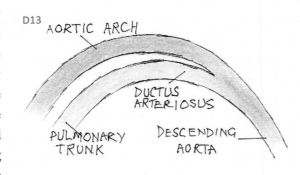

representation of it after birth, when the ductus has closed and shrunk. The ductus was a large vessel, as large as the aorta, and the two vessels lay side by side with a narrow angle between them, converging to form the beginning of the descending aorta. D 13.

What are we to make of these findings?

1)  They confirm what I have said earlier that the upper part of the inferior vena cava carrying blood from the placenta enters the left atrium.

2)  Venous blood from the superior vena cava enters the right atrium.

3)  The ductus arteriosus does not enter the aorta.

4)  We still do not know the path taken by the venous flow in the lower part of the inferior vena cava. But it cannot join the placental flow, either separated by streaming or as part of a mixed homogeneous stream, and therefore *must take an alternative route.*

In May 1967 I was posted from Fort Victoria to Salisbury, which is now called Harare, and worked mainly in the large Harare Hospital. This turned out to be a very good move with many benefits for the family, and for me a deeper understanding of the foetal circulation. Saturday morning clinical meetings were held in Harare hospital and I gave four presentations: the first on 24th February 1968 was about my observations on the foetal heart. It led to my being invited to examine human foetuses in our medical school.

D14

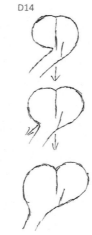

The first thing I did in the anatomy department, was to examine a foetal right atrium and look for the inferior vena cava attached to the septum round the foramen ovale. But I did not find it; the vena cava led into the right atrium, as it does in the postnate. Without doubt it was a foetus because it had not breathed, and the thoracic organs were closely packed together in the foetal condition. In the other specimens I examined I found the same arrangement. The right atrium in each of these specimens must have unrolled spontaneously either in utero or afterwards, and I presume that at the moment of death, without a cardiac impulse from the pacemaker, the flaccid right atrium may have fallen away from the septum and revealed the postnatal position. D 14. In which case the other investigators could have been forgiven for assuming that the inferior vena cava led into the right atrium.

I turned my attention to the foramen ovale and found that it was not a 'little flap valve' as described in some accounts. The name means an oval hole, but when we talk about it, we mean the hole and the parts which cover the hole, the 'whole' thing. It consists of two septa: primum and secundum guarding the entrance to the left atrium like the Pillars of Hercules, fused together below and separated above, movement between them allowing blood to pass into the left atrium. The oval hole is the cut-out part of septum secundum facing the right atrium, covered by septum primum facing the left atrium. D 15.

D15

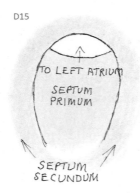

TO LEFT ATRIUM

SEPTUM PRIMUM

SEPTUM SECUNDUM

I have three drawings of the valve made in 1968. 'A' shows the valve in the medial wall of the right atrium. 'B' shows the interior of the left atrium, with the atrioventricular opening on the left and the valve on the right. 'C' gives a good view of septum primum in the medial wall of the left atrium, with the upper part of secundum beyond.

It would seem obvious from these drawings that the blood entering the left atrium would have come from the right atrium, but with the atria beating together at the same time there could not have been a flow between them. The authors of the orthodox accounts may have recognised this difficulty, because they say the blood flows through, passes through or is shunted through from high pressure in the right atrium to lower pressure in the left atrium; even though the valve would seem to be designed to prevent backflow from a higher pressure in the left atrium. Now we see the importance of my findings in that little girl's heart, which showed the inferior vena cava covering the valve in the atrial septum and leading the placental flow directly into the left atrium without entering the right atrium at all.

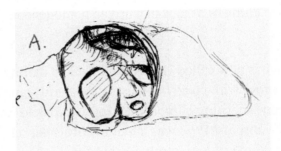 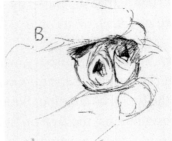 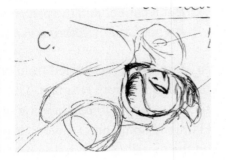

During my work at the medical school I kept my drawings made in 1965 in a nearby cupboard. They disappeared and I do not have a permanent record of my original findings; my diagrams of them here have been made from memory.

I paid a visit to the library of our University Veterinary School. I wanted to see if mammals other than the human had a foramen ovale and musculi pectinati. I thought they must have, but I wanted to confirm it. I read books on the anatomy of the horse, dog and pig. Each one of them had those two features, but there was a third structure common to all of them and to the human. I wondered why those 'lower' creatures should have what we have in our anatomy; was it important? Then I realised its true function in the foetal circulation of us all. *It was the azygos vein.* This vessel connects the two venae cavae and *would serve as the alternative pathway* for the lower venous return to reach the right atrium through the superior vena cava, if the inferior vena cava is blocked to prevent contamination of the arterial stream for the left atrium. D 16.

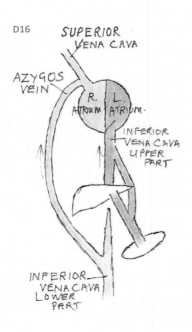

No one would deny the importance of the foramen ovale in allowing the placental stream to enter the left atrium. But what about the other feature never mentioned in the orthodox accounts which I read about in the Veterinary School Library: the musculi pectinati? Are they not important? Let us have a look at them. The right atrium is in two parts: a smooth upper part developed from the primitive sinus venosus, and a lower muscular part containing the musculi pectinati originating in the primitive atrium. Blood is collected in the smooth part and pumped into the right ventricle by the muscular part. The musculi seem to be an integral part of the pumping mechanism. In the postnate the total venous return enters the right atrium through two venae cavae at a relatively low rate of about seventy beats per minute. But in the foetus, if I am correct about the alternative pathway, the superior vena cava would carry the total return at twice that speed, and in the rolled up shape of the right atrium the musculi would be closer together and form a more efficient pump to manage this part of the circulation, with perhaps the more subsidiary role of aiding the flow in the postnate. If the superior vena cava does carry all the venous return to the right atrium, it would be one of the reasons for the fast foetal heart rate; there may be others. The musculi pectinati are important; upon their healthy functioning depends the future of the human race, and of all those other creatures which possess them.

At the end of 1969 I resigned from the government medical service, and in April the following year opened my own medical practice in the Harare suburb of Greendale, leaving the university work and putting off further investigation of the foetus till another day. This came much later than I had expected, and in 2004, when I had become an octogenarian and my practice had become quieter, it began to occupy my mind more and more. In 2011 I produced my own little book. The observations were valuable; some of my opinions questionable. But it was a start, and if I had not begun then I might not have reached the present position, where I have been able to explore and develop my ideas further. In 2013 Pauline died, and I returned to England, where I have continued to write new versions of my book. What I need to make my work more acceptable and to follow up on the work I had begun in Africa, is to examine more human foetuses, but this has been denied me. However, I have been fortunate in being able to make other important observations, as I will shortly reveal.

Since finding the foetal heart in the mortuary I had believed that it is the *foetus* which is delivered, and that the foetus changes into a baby *after* the delivery when the first deep breath is taken. I was therefore very interested in a programme on television which showed the birth of a foal, and I followed it very carefully. At first, the non-breathing lifeless-looking form of the animal with a narrow unexpanded chest, was delivered on to the ground. Then almost immediately it took a deep breath, opened its chest, stood up on all four legs and shook itself. My belief was confirmed; I had seen a foetus change into a foal. In another programme on television I watched the delivery of a goat kid. It emerged in a flaccid lifeless form and did not breathe. It was still born, and I knew I had watched the delivery of a foetus.

I then realised that stillborn farm animals could be a valuable source of information on the foetal circulation if human foetuses were unavailable, and in February 2018, during the lambing season, Graham Jones, a sheep farmer near Oswestry, kindly gave me four stillborn lambs. (Two were very haemorrhagic, one of them dripping with blood. The previous summer had been long and dry, with little fresh grazing for the farm animals which had been fed with stored fodder. The two had probably died from spoiled sweet clover disease). The little 'girl' in the mortuary had not been stillborn; she had been delivered alive and had died afterwards. Hers was therefore a neonatal death, but it is the failure to breathe which is common to both the stillborn and the apnoeic neonatal death, and in each case the circulation would not have changed from the foetal to that of a baby.

In the lambing season of 2019, I was able to examine two more foetal lambs, again supplied by Graham Jones. I examined the whole length of an inferior vena cava and could not find a block or an azygos vein. However, in the human foetus and in the horse, dog and pig there is an azygos vein, and I presume there are other alternative routes for the lower return to reach the right atrium in the foetal lamb. In which case the inferior vena cava would be divided into two sections: the lower to carry the lower venous return to the right atrium, and the upper to carry the placental stream to the left atrium. Strictly speaking the upper section should not be called a vena cava because it carries arterial blood to the left atrium and should be given a new name.

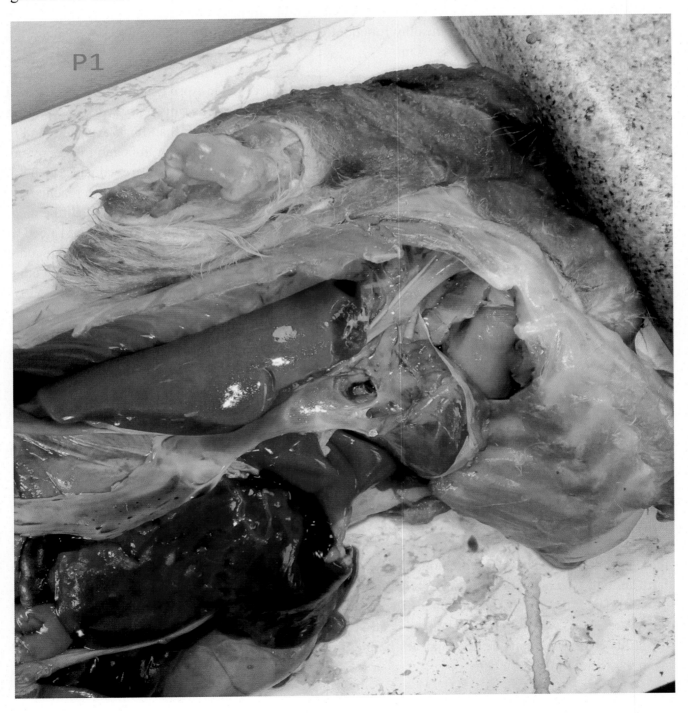

The above picture, P1, from a foetal lamb, taken with my mobile phone camera and which I have enlarged, is very revealing: it shows clearly all the details of this section of the circulation. Branching off the inferior vena cava just before it reaches the foramen ovale is a channel leading to the right atrium, which has been opened, and shows the end of the channel above the opening of the coronary sinus. Between these two features is a crescentic blade which probably helps to convert each into a valve and prevent backflow in atrial systole. D 17 helps to explain.

This pre-terminal branch of the inferior vena cava is very important, it is in effect an arterio-venous fistula providing oxygen and food for the respiratory capillaries of the foetal lungs. In the postnate the capillaries of the respiratory zone are the first to receive oxygen from the air in the closely adjacent lung airways, but the non-functional foetal lungs have no access to air. This branch provides them with oxygen and food from the placental stream in the inferior vena cava, which leads blood not only to the right atrium, right ventricle and the pulmonary trunk, but to the pulmonary arteries and the respiratory capillaries in the respiratory zone. It is an unusual arrangement for the lungs, with the pulmonary arteries bringing in oxygen instead of carbon di-oxide, and the pulmonary veins returning to the left atrium with carbon di-oxide instead of oxygen. Without this branch there would be no lungs, no people, no mammals, and perhaps no birds. This branch and its terminal valve deserve names. D 18. (When the blood passes through the right atrium it will also pick up Co2 from the superior vena cava, which will be carried with the oxygen and food to the respiratory zone).

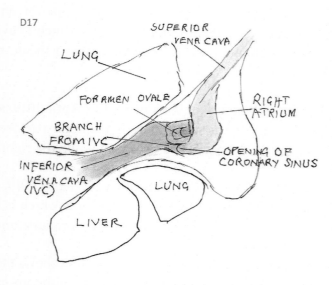

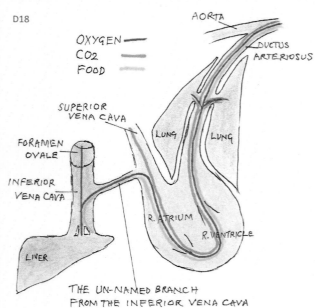

Interestingly, the Oxford team had identified this unnamed stream. Referring back to the sentence, part of which I have already quoted, they say 'In addition, however, a certain quantity is detached from the mainstream in the right auricle and is carried through the right atrio-ventricular (tricuspid) valve to the right ventricle and pulmonary trunk. Hence, we see a relatively faint shadow in the right side of the heart and pulmonary arteries, *i.e.,* the flow is comparatively small in relation to the mainstream through the left side of the heart and aortic valve.' (The 'certain quantity' is not detached *in* the right atrium, it is detached from the mainstream inferior vena cava and then *enters* the right atrium).

In another article from the British Journal of Radiology, Vol XV, No. 177, by A. E. Barclay, K. J. Franklin and M. M. L. Prichard, the authors have introduced their own names for two structures: the *crista dividens* and the *crista interveniens*. The first refers to the 'V' shaped branching of the vessel from the inferior vena cava, while the second appears to refer to the crescentic blade between the end of this vessel and the opening of the coronary sinus.

There are four more pictures here, also taken with my mobile phone camera. The first P2, was taken on 7th June 2018. The longer stick is in the superior vena cava leading into the right atrium, while the short stick props open the inferior vena cava, which I have cut, and which leads to the foramen ovale at the far end. Branching off the inferior vena cava is the un-named vessel which leads into the right atrium above the opening of the coronary sinus.

The second picture, P3, taken on 22nd April 2019, shows the inferior vena cava, which I have cut open, branching at the crista dividens into a larger part feeding the foramen ovale on the left, and a smaller part which is the un-named vessel leading into the right atrium on the right.

The third picture, P4, also taken on 22nd April 2019, does not show the crista dividens so clearly, but gives an excellent view of the crescentic blade, which is the crista interveniens, separating the end of the un-named vessel from the opening of the coronary sinus into the right atrium.

The last picture, P5, taken on 7th July 2018, shows the scar of the foramen ovale, known as the fossa ovalis, in a postnatal lamb. It includes the scar of the un-named vessel on its right side, which is best seen with a magnifying glass.

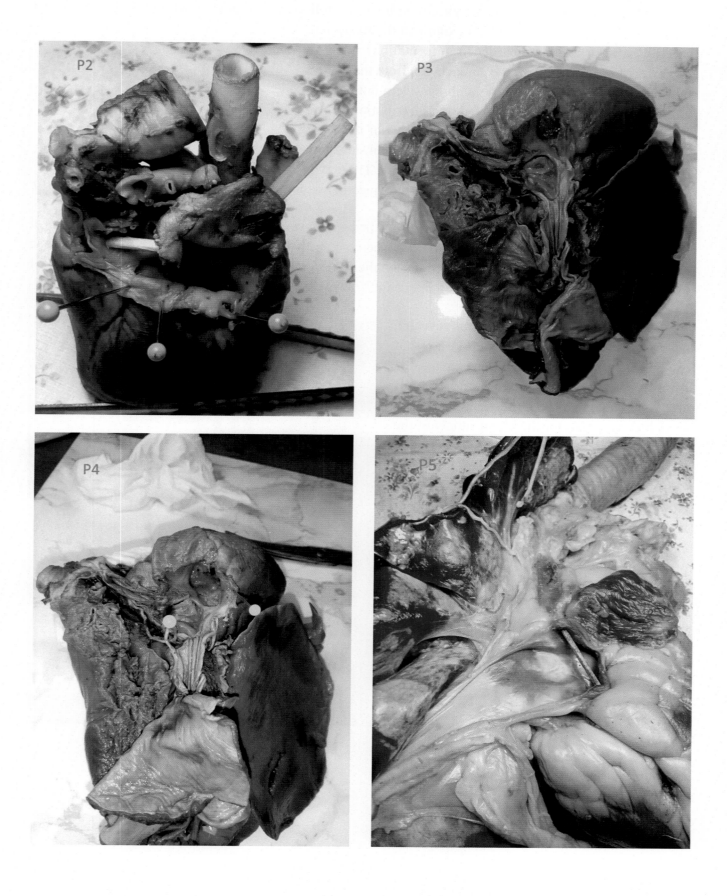

In 2018 I had traced the umbilical vein to the liver and followed its branches within the liver, without finding a ductus venosus. In 2019 I examined the liver more carefully after it had been hardened in formalin. I spent all day meticulously picking off the parenchyma from the vessels with my dissecting forceps. The umbilical vein entered the left side of the liver. It then arrived at a distribution centre from where branches spread out to every part of the liver. There was a large branch leading across to the right side, with smaller branches being given off along the way. There was another large branch leading to the south west, connecting with the portal vein near the gall bladder. D 19.

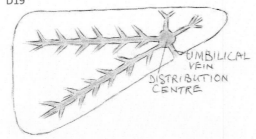

I started to uncover the tributaries and trunks of the hepatic veins. There were two large main trunks at the top edge of the liver, with a smaller one between them; I had severed them all from the inferior vena cava when I removed the liver. I followed the smaller one down and traced it to the distribution centre. I exposed the whole channel cleanly then opened it. *It was the ductus venosus inside the liver.* P6.

My examination of the foetal lambs revealed several features. a) It confirmed again that the upper part of the inferior vena cava leads directly to the foramen ovale and the left atrium. b) It identified the pre-terminal branch from the vena cava for the blood supply of the lungs. c) It demonstrated the distribution of the placental blood supply for the foetal liver. d) It showed how the ductus venosus within the liver carries the placental stream into the inferior vena cava. I have proposed that the upper vena cava should be given a new name, and that its pre-terminal branch and valve should be given names. Once the names have been given, much of the confusion which has surrounded this part of the foetal circulation for so long will have disappeared, but a picture or a diagram such as the ones I have given will always be a helpful accompaniment.

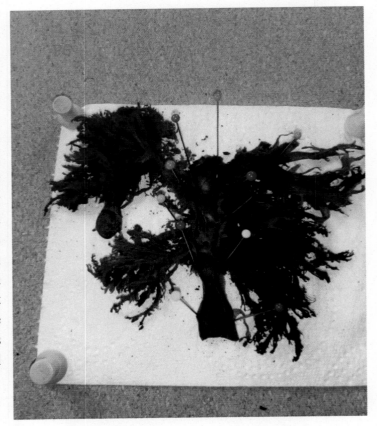

We can now make a plan of the foetal circulation, with the upper and lower returns leading to the right atrium and the placental stream leading to the left atrium. D 20.

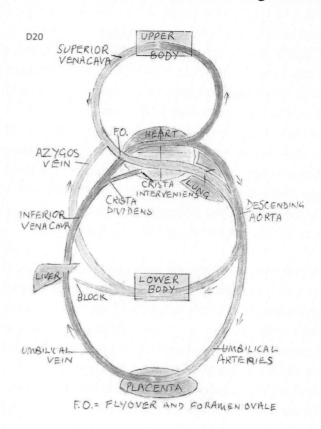

D20

F.O. = FLYOVER AND FORAMEN OVALE

Note the terminal venous flow in the umbilical arteries to the placenta which will be explained in my account of the placental circulation.

In D 21, I have introduced a different plan of the circulation which separates the heart into its two sides. They are normally joined as one because the right side shares the coronary arterial supply from the left, the coronary venous drainage of the left empties into the right, and both share the impulses from the pacemaker in the right atrium.

I have again separated the foetus into upper and lower parts and shown the alternative route as the azygos vein. I have not shown the un-named vessel supplying some arterial blood to the right atrium, or the return from the lungs supplying some venous blood to the left atrium. Otherwise I think the plan is complete. Although the blood stream in the descending aorta is mixed homogeneous, I have separated the component parts into arterial and venous. We know from direct

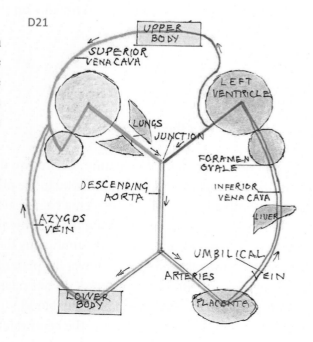

D21

observation of the junction that the arterial and venous flows in the descending aorta are approximately equal and large. This would mean that the arterial and venous flows to the lower body would be equal, and the mixed flows to the placenta would also be equal. The total blood supply to the foetus is divided between mainly pure arterial for the upper body and mixed homogeneous for the lower body, with the total venous return entering the right atrium and ventricle. Clearly seen is the path taken by this total venous return from the right heart to the placenta. The amount reaching the placenta must equal the total return from the foetus or the circulation would not be sustainable. The venous supply for the lower body would therefore be an additional supply which has not participated in the metabolism of the foetus, except for a small flow from the lungs. It would seem likely, therefore, that the venous return in the azygos vein would include an appreciable and equal additional amount as well as the venous return from the metabolism of the lower body. The increased return to the right atrium would join the mainstream leaving the right ventricle and re-circulate to the lower body indefinitely. We can easily see that the mixed flow to the placenta would be far greater than the mixed flow to the lower body: the placental flow equates to twice the arterial supply to the foetus, while the other equals twice the arterial supply for the lower body.

The total disposal of the carbon dioxide ($CO_2$), has therefore two pathways: the major one from the foetal body to the placenta and a minor one to the lower body which is the additional supply carrying the venous return from the lungs. The latter will equate to the oxygen supplied to the lungs from the inferior vena cava at the crista dividens, and the $CO_2$ leaving the lungs in the pulmonary veins will pass through the left atrium and contaminate the arterial supply for the upper body before reaching the mixed stream in the descending aorta. The venous blood returning from the lower body consists of two equal portions: from the metabolism of the lower body and the additional supply. The arterial blood returning from the placenta also consists of two equal portions: one from the metabolism of the foetus and the other from the metabolism of the placenta. One can now see why the foetal heart, at 140 beats per minute, beats twice as quickly as the postnate at 70: it accommodates twice as much blood; half for the foetus and half for the placenta. After birth when the placenta has been jettisoned, the rate will slow, and other factors will come into play. cf. supra, see my comments on the increased speed in the superior vena cava.

Part Two.

## The Sections.

The Circulation for the Placenta.

The Junction is a remarkable feature, where two different streams of similar size meet and send mixed blood to the placenta and lower body. The mixed stream for the placenta begins in the internal iliac arteries, and branching off them are the umbilical arteries, which ascend on the abdominal wall to the umbilicus then travel outside the foetus to the placenta. D 22 shows the plan of the vessels but is misleading, the umbilical arteries do not pass downwards. D 23 is more accurate and shows how the blood will circulate. The dotted uncoloured circle represents the central left atrium behind the right heart.

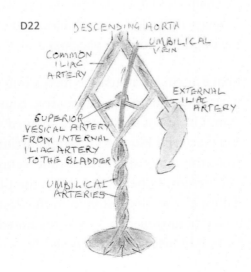

The plan of the foetal circulation we have inherited is similar to that of the baby and is just as beautifully simple. But it has been represented falsely as ugly and complicated. *It is the similarity of the simple designs of the foetus and the baby which allows the one to change into the other at the moment of birth.*

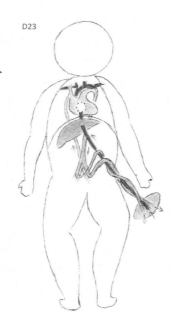

The placenta is in two parts: a foetal part which receives the umbilical arteries and a maternal part supplied by the uterine arteries, with the interface between them across which the respiratory gases, food and waste can pass in solution. The fact that the placenta has an arterial blood supply with oxygen and food, indicates that it has work to do, if it wasn't obvious already, and it seems appropriate that the arterial stream should be of similar size to the venous to provide the necessary energy for the purification. As the oxygen of the mixed stream passes through the umbilical arteres and the placenta, it would be used up in producing the energy and replaced by carbon-dioxide, *and all the blood reaching the interface would be venous.* The maternal side would then receive the carbon-dioxide and waste and give in return to the umbilical vein oxygen and food: half for the foetus and the umbilical vein, and half for the placenta and the umbilical arteries; probably as quickly as the respiratory exchanges in the boat race crews.

The Venturi/ Segregation.

I had often driven through a road junction in Harare where two lanes of traffic converged into one, and the speed of the vehicles in the single lane ahead was twice the speed of the double stream behind. D 24.

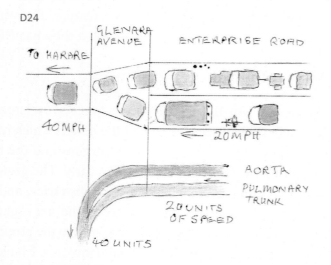

This reminded me of the junction in the foetus where two streams joined into one, and I assumed the speed of the blood flowing down the descending aorta after the junction would be twice as fast as the speed in each of the streams meeting at the junction. This is part of the Venturi Principle or Effect, which concerns the increased speed and lowered pressure in a stream of liquid flowing through a narrow section of a tube. (Giovanni Venturi 1797). The junction would therefore segregate the blood supply of the upper body of the foetus coming off the aorta before the junction, from the supply for the lower body and placenta coming off the descending aorta. That for the upper body would be at high pressure, with a full complement of oxygen and food, low in carbon-dioxide and waste (if any), flowing at a certain speed. The mixed stream beyond the junction for the lower body and placenta would be at lower pressure, with less oxygen and food, an increased amount of carbon dioxide and waste, flowing faster than the other.

On 30th March 2019 I removed part of the second lamb which I had kept in formalin, and with my mini Vernier calliper measured the diameters of the vessels before and after the junction. The aorta before the junction measured 22mm, the pulmonary trunk 20.6mm and the descending aorta 26.6mm. The corresponding cross section areas would have been, aorta 363 square mm, pulmonary trunk 318 square mm, and descending aorta 530 square mm. The total area of the aorta and trunk before the junction would have been 681 sq.mm, and the reduction of area in the descending aorta 151 sq.mm. This is a reduction of 22.17%, and perhaps the increase in speed would be a similar figure. Formalin distorted the vessels; I should have measured them before I had preserved them; the results then may have been more reliable.

## The Circulation for the Upper Body.

### D 25.

The upper body of the human foetus is supplied by three arteries, apart from the coronary arteries for the heart. In the lamb there is only one, which I have called 'cephalic.' The Oxford team called it brachiocephalic,' which is more appropriate, because it feeds the forelimbs as well as the head and neck. The arteries in each case come off the aortic arch between the flyover and the junction. It is the most important part of the circulation for the foetus, with a rich supply of oxygen relatively free from carbon-dioxide, which shows the importance

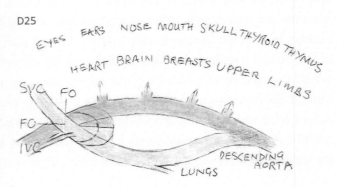

FO=Flyover & Foramen Ovale SVC = Superior vena cava IVC = Inferior vena cava

of them in the assembly of the new creature. The venous return from the upper body flows in the superior vena cava to the right atrium, as I have shown earlier.

## The Circulation for the Lower Body.

We can see why the placenta needs to receive a large flow of venous blood, but why should the lower body have a portion? I see it as part of the design which reduces the size of the lower body and the development of the abdominal viscera, the sex organs and the lower limbs, while allowing the heart, the head, the brain and the upper limbs to mature early. The gestation period is also reduced, the head is better shaped and better prepared for the delivery obstetrics, and the hands will be needed early to adjust to the new environment. The abdominal viscera, the sex organs and legs can develop later after birth. Without the venous blood supply, the foetus might have the proportions of an adult, with the mother carrying a monster unable to navigate the birth canal. However, I have not considered the position of the foetal lambs and other quadrupeds which run around with their mothers shortly after birth, with early development of their hind legs, in spite of a 50/50 mixed blood supply. There must be something else to consider.

The venous return from the upper part of the lower body probably travels in the hemiazygos system to the right atrium, while most of the lower return would be diverted in the azygos vein and join the upper return entering the right atrium from the superior vena cava.

The Junction.

The junction is more than remarkable, it is astonishing, where two quite different blood streams use the same vessel. In the realms of anatomy and physiology it is entirely new and unique, (apart from the arterio-venous fistula mentioned earlier). But don't forget what I said about homo sapiens when we were first planted on this earth. Are we not reminded that we were divinely made to last, long long ago? Whether you believe this or not, only a supreme genius would have been able to design it so, (with all the other parts too). It cuts out the need to make an extra vessel which would have had to be dismantled at birth. It ensures that the foetus is timely matured and perfectly designed for good obstetrics at birth and ensures that the energy for the placenta is right where it is needed when the venous blood is carried to the interface. There may be hidden reasons too, but it works, and has done so from the beginning. The postnatal circulation consists of a large part for the body and the smaller pulmonary. In the foetus the larger part is the mixed supply for the placenta and lower body, the smaller part is the arterial supply for the upper body.

The junction has been misunderstood and could not have been seen by some of those who have described it. It is often shown with the ductus entering the aorta at a right angle or almost a right angle, and sometimes the ductus is smaller than the aorta, D 26.

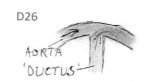

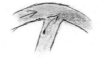

What I saw in 1965 was quite different, as I said earlier. Both vessels were large, of the same size and lay side by side with a small angle between them. They converged together and merged into a single vessel that was the descending aorta. Now we must be quite clear on this point; *neither vessel enters the other.* They lie side by side almost like the twin barrels of a double-barrelled shot gun and *enter the descending aorta together.* D.27.

The two vessels are derivatives of the primitive aortic arches: the aorta from the 4th arch and the pulmonary trunk from the 6th. (The 5th arches are said to disappear completely, but I suspect they may have developed into the two coronary arteries). D 28.

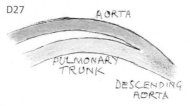

After birth, when the ductus is called the ligamentum arteriosum, the ligamentum does look like a ductus and suggests there would have been a shunt, but in the foetus, there is neither. D 29. *The concept of a ductus arteriosus leading into the aorta is a complete myth;* the primitive arches were never connected like this. However, it needs a name and it is best to retain it, providing that those who do so understand that it lies at the side of the aorta and does not enter it.

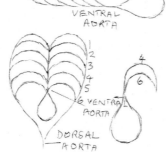

## The Foramen Ovale.

After birth when the foramen ovale has closed, it becomes converted into a scar known as the fossa ovalis, which lies in the septum between the two atria. It has bedevilled us for ages and has suggested that in the foetus, the arterial oxygenated blood from the placenta in the inferior vena cava entered the right atrium and passed through the valve into the left atrium. It could not be pumped through, because the two atria beating together in time on either side of the septum would not be able to propel it through. So it was assumed, as I mentioned earlier in part one, that the pressure in the right atrium was greater than the pressure in the left atrium, and that the blood passed through, entered through, flowed through, was directed through or shunted through; without consideration of the structure of the valve, which appeared to be designed to prevent backflow from a higher pressure in the left atrium to a lower pressure in the right. It was a paradox, an enigma, a riddle unsolved until the death of that little girl in April 1965 which showed that the stream from the placenta in the inferior vena cava led into the *left* atrium, not the right.

The foetal heart has five valves, one more than the postnate, the extra one being the foramen ovale. It is an inlet valve, the only pure inlet valve of the heart. The atrio-ventricular valves are mixed: outlet for the atria and inlet for the ventricles. I believe inlet valves are opened actively by the muscles attached to them, while outlet valves are opened passively by the weight of the blood pushing the cusps aside. In the condition of atrial fibrillation, the ventricles get little or no help from the atria, and the ventricles do all the work pumping the blood through the heart. The atrio-ventricular valves, without the atrial component, then become pure inlet valves, opening actively in ventricular diastole, as well as closing actively in ventricular systole. Every person walking around with atrial fibrillation, including myself, is living proof of the ventricles working in ventricular diastole; we cannot live without it. We therefore must abandon the concept of the heart muscles working only in systole and relaxing in diastole. There must be two sets of heart muscle closely apposed: one to contract in ventricular systole while the other relaxes, and the other to contract in ventricular diastole while the first relaxes. Perhaps we may have to reconsider the interpretation of the electrocardiogram. Could the biphasic RS component be due to the double muscular action I have just described? Atrial fibrillation, abbreviated to AF, is a pathological condition, said to affect the atria. I have not heard of it affecting only one atrium, and I presume that the fault may therefore lie in the pacemaker rather than in the atria.

My own AF began when I was 45, sprinting after one of my children in the garden. Suddenly there was a gobble gobble gobble in the left side of my chest which brought me to a standstill. I think a large surge of blood from my leg veins had dilated the right atrium. It settled down to a normal rhythm in a few days. It happened a second time 30 years later when I was sprinting across a bowling green, chasing my wood. There was the gobble gobble gobble again followed by AF which has been with me ever since. In 2013, shortly after returning to England, I developed complete heart block and was given a pacemaker. This was a good combination because I need not take digitalis to reduce the rate of the atrial beats; no beats reach the ventricles.

An inlet valve opens in diastole to admit a measured amount of blood and closes in systole to prevent backflow and eject the blood forwards. If we consider the two atria of the foetal heart and the two atria of the postnatal heart, prevention of backflow in atrial systole will be helped in all four by the action of the ventricles in diastole which I have just described, which sucks the blood forward. The foramen ovale, being an inlet valve, will also strongly prevent backflow from the foetal left atrium when it closes. But the other three atria without inlet valves must prevent backflow in other ways. In the postnatal and foetal right atria it would be important for the sensors of the pacemaker mechanism to have unobstructed access to the venous return from the body. An inlet valve at the entrance to the atrium might be an impediment, and perhaps as a compensating feature is the collection of the six valves in the jugular and subclavian veins preventing backflow from the right atrium to the head and neck and the upper limbs. D 30. Also, the milking mechanism which I have described would have a valve-like action, helping to propel the blood forwards.

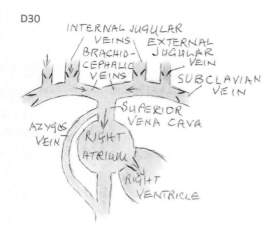

With the postnatal left atrium, I have considered two factors. The first is the bellows-like action of the lungs, taking in air and blood in inspiration and forcing them out in expiration, expiration taking longer than inspiration. Then there is the backup power of the right ventricle nearby which pumps a continuous flow of venous blood to the lungs throughout the cardiac cycle. But I had overlooked some of my own

work which I had carried out in the anatomy department of our medical school. I made several drawings there. One of them, drawing D, with several interesting features, is very informative. IA and IV are abbreviations for the innominate artery and vein, now called brachiocephalic. A represents the aorta, DA the ductus arteriosus, PA's the pulmonary arteries, PV's the pulmonary veins, and IVC and SVC are the two venae cavae. I have removed the heart from the vessels which pass through the parietal pericardium. The roughly drawn line round the entrances of the pulmonary veins is where the left atrium would have been

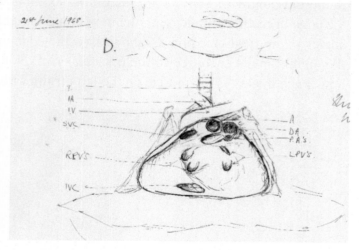

attached, and we are looking at the openings of the pulmonary veins which lead into the left atrium. Three of the openings are oblique and would appear to indicate a valve-like action, preventing backflow into the veins in atrial systole. (The fourth cannot be seen properly). This would apply not only in the foetus when there is a small flow of venous blood from the pulmonary veins into the atrium, but in the neonate too, when all the large inflow from the lungs would be arterial. (The foetus has helped us to understand the postnate; there are other examples elsewhere). The position of the inferior vena cava shows that the foramen ovale in the wall of the atrium would have been situated close to the lower right pulmonary vein. Five veins and their valves would have been functioning to bring blood into the left atrium: the four pulmonary veins bringing in a trickle of venous blood, and the inferior vena cava and foramen ovale bringing in a large single stream of arterial blood. The flow through the foramen ovale in the foetus would have been as large as the combined arterial flows through the pulmonary veins of the neonate at the moment of birth. The foramen ovale must be a strong structure made to last, not only in the foetus as a valve to prevent backflow, but after birth *for as long as the life of the owner,* when the two septa will be fused together as the fossa ovalis and separate the two atria. Also, it must be smooth, without any encumbrances such as chordae tendinae, to affect the flows of blood through the postnatal atria.

On 22nd April 2019 I investigated the foramen ovale from a foetal lamb which had been kept in 10% formalin. I opened the left atrium and looked at the valve carefully from both sides. Round the periphery on each side was a ring of thickened tissue, and the valve membrane was attached to it. The top part of the membrane was thickened and anchored at each end, and crescentic in shape leaving a gap above. It was a loose membrane which could be distended but not stretched, like a ship's sail which billows out in the wind. I tried to work out how the valve would have functioned. In atrial diastole, P7, the membrane would have ballooned inwards towards the left atrium, allowing blood to flow through the crescentic gap into the atrium. Then in systole, P8, it would have ballooned the other way, pushing the membrane against the atrial wall, closing the gap between the crescent and the ring and preventing backflow into the inferior vena cava.

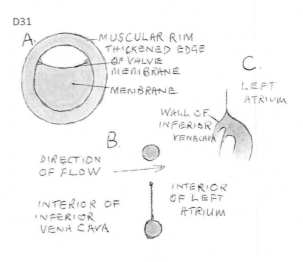

D 31 gives three views of the valve. A. gives a complete view from either side, showing the membrane attached to the muscular rim. In B., I am imagining looking at the edge of the membrane, with the membrane at right angles to my field of vision. C. shows how the edge of the membrane is anchored to the muscular rim. Note how much thicker is the muscle on the left atrium side.

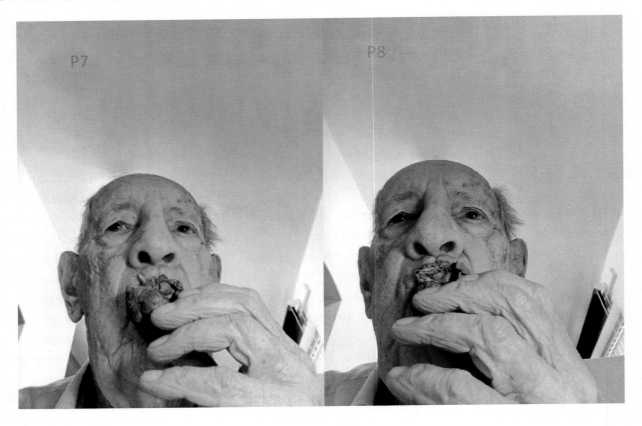

The next day I blew onto the valve from each side, looking into a mirror held on the opposite side of the valve. When I blew from the vena cava side, P7, I could see the membrane ballooning out beyond the valve, with air escaping easily through the crescentic gap, as blood would have entered the left atrium in atrial diastole. When I blew from the left atrium side, P8, the membrane ballooned out into the inferior vena cava side, as it would have done in atrial systole, but the air did not escape through the valve, it escaped outside the valve, on each side across my lips. I then fetched my mobile phone and repeated the blowing onto the valve from both sides, taking pictures with the camera. I enjoyed looking at the pictures, except for my ugly nose of course; it isn't the one I was born with. In May 1961 on a lonely Nyasaland road in the middle of the night, returning to Lilongwe from a court case in Blantyre, I was assaulted by a thug, who clobbered me and knocked me out cold. He damaged my nose and I could not breathe through it properly. A few weeks later I was back in England on home leave. I did not tell my parents about the assault, but while I was sitting in the garden my mother came up to me looking very concerned. She told me how she had woken suddenly in the night a few weeks earlier, sat up and woken my father and said: 'something's happened to Alan.' I had surgery on my nose, and I looked like a rugby player or a boxer who had had a similar operation. I was wrong to blow from the vena cava side; I should have sucked from the left atrium side, to copy what happens in the foetus in atrial diastole. I wanted to do this, again with my camera at the ready, but I could not find the specimen; I must have disposed of it - foolishly.

I investigated the valve further. It had been distorted somewhat by the formalin. The diameter was about 10mm., and the length of the crescentic gap 3mm. I wanted to confirm that the ring/rim of thickened tissue surrounding the membrane was muscle, so I fetched my microscope and examined a small piece; first at times 40, then at times 100, and lastly at times 400 magnifications. The tissue was unstained of course, and a bit dry, but I could easily make out the parallel strips of tissue which ran across my field of vision in a somewhat wavy fashion. I scrutinised them even more carefully and at the highest magnification eventually found some of the strips with barely visible tiny transverse striations. It was muscle: without doubt cardiac! But how would it have functioned during the beating of the left atrium? As I have said previously there must be two sets of cardiac muscle functioning together: one to contract the ring and close the valve in systole, and the other to dilate the ring and suck in blood in diastole. (Somatic muscle is different: the two sets are the protagonists and the antagonists in separate groups of muscle).

There are four pictures here, the first, P9, showing the foramen ovale of a foetal lamb at the end of the opened inferior vena cava. The second picture, P10, shows the valve from the left atrium side. In the third picture, P11, I have removed the valve, and again viewed it from the left atrium side. The last picture P12, shows the valve from inside the inferior vena cava. From my examination of the foramen ovale I could see that there was more muscle on the left atrium side, but this increase of muscle is not so evident in these pictures. However, the muscle would have been part of the left atrial wall and supports what I have said that the left atrium controls the flow of blood into the atrium, rather than being dependent on the inflow, as has been alleged by the orthodox.

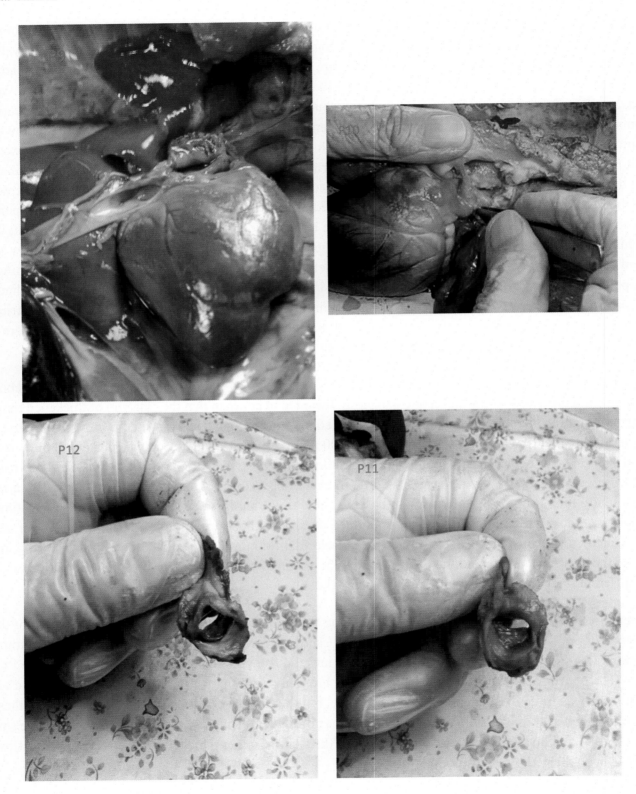

Since having examined and drawn the human foramen ovale in the medical school, I had believed that the valve would be an active one, more likely to control the blood flow, rather than a passive little flap blown hither and thither by the blood stream. My examination of the valve of the foetal lamb has confirmed these ideas, but in some of my diagrams in part one I have shown the valve as a little flap, only to represent it as a valve.

The Left Atrium.

We can learn more from drawing D. The heart almost fills the whole chest and the unexpanded lungs lie at the sides and behind the heart. Sometimes the foetal lungs are said to be collapsed. They are not collapsed, they are unexpanded. Collapse is a pathological condition which affects the expanded lungs after birth.

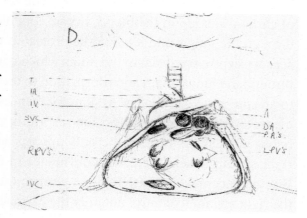

Note the difference between the circular muscular aorta and ductus, and the flattened venae cavae. The pulmonary arteries arise from the pulmonary trunk proximal to the ductus, so what I have called the ductus is really part of the trunk. It is as large as the aorta and lies by the side of the aorta without any indication of leading into it. We are never given a good view of the left atrium; it is a central posterior structure of the heart with only the auricle on the left side. But it is not only a central part of the heart; it is the central part of the circulation in the foetus and the baby. That is why I have illustrated it in an unusual way in my diagrams.

In the drawing we see the trachea and the right main bronchus branching from it. What we cannot see is the oesophagus which runs down the neck behind the trachea. After the branching of the main bronchi the oesophagus continues to pass down behind the left atrium to the stomach; it forms a bed on which the left atrium lies. Do we not see therefore, why we are given a hot drink when we come in out of the cold, warming the blood in the left atrium as it is delivered to every part of the body, especially the cold feet? Whisky must work in a different way, by vasodilation, and a hot toddy would work both ways. And do we not enjoy the cooling by a large ice-cream as it passes down behind the left atrium, on the beach on a hot summer's day? (*Hot toddy: a hot lemon drink with sugar and whisky*).

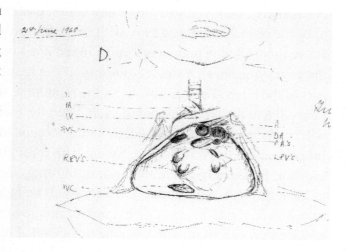

I have devoted the previous two sections to the foramen ovale and the left atrium; they are inseparable and require further comment. I am bringing in drawing D for a third time because it is the most important of the illustrations I have made and will make. It is a precious drawing, made as you can see, on the 21st of June 1968. It does not show the foramen ovale; it had been taken away when I removed the heart. But it does reveal the function of the valve; it is staring us in the face. Do we not see the pulmonary valves which will ensure a constant supply of oxygenated blood for the left atrium at birth? And will not the foramen ovale have the same function for the foetal left atrium? You may forget all I have written and will write, but please remember that *the function of the foramen ovale is to ensure a constant supply of oxygenated blood for the left atrium*. It has absolutely nothing to do with shunting blood from one side of the heart to the other.

For the time being we must say goodbye to this shy recluse. We will meet it again in the third and fourth sections.

## The Postnatal Right Atrium.

I have found it difficult to accept that the respiratory centre in the brain stem could analyse the level of carbon-dioxide in the blood, because its blood supply would have been purified already by passage through the lungs, and it would be protected from the toxic effects of the CO2. I think there must be a sensory centre proximal to the lungs which can detect the levels of CO2 in the blood before it has passed through the lungs and relay information to the respiratory centre, which could adjust the respiratory rate to an appropriate level. The system for respiratory control would then consist of three parts: the sensory centre proximal to the lungs, the respiratory centre distal to the lungs, with the lungs in the middle between each. As I see it, the only appropriate place for the detection of the CO2 levels would be the right atrium, where there is a confluence of all the venous blood arriving from the peripheral tissues. But the pacemaker controlling the cardiac output is also in the right atrium. Is it possible therefore for the right atrium to control not only the cardiac output, but the respiratory rate as well? In which case any activity of the body would be matched by comparable increases in the heart and respiratory rates, under the eventual control of the cardiac and respiratory centres in the brain stem.

## The Lungs.

In 1953 I visited the John Hunter Museum in the Royal College of Surgeons in London and saw two beautiful casts of the lungs. The bronchi and pulmonary vessels had been injected with resin and the other tissues had been removed with acid. I noticed a pattern in the relationship between the bronchi and the vessels, but there was no description of it nearby. I have not seen another description of the pattern I had noticed, so I am now describing what I saw in 1953. If you take a key ring and hold it out horizontally, then you can pull a key out on each side. Imagine the keys to be the bronchi painted green, with the pulmonary arteries in blue lying above them and the pulmonary veins in red lying below. Without twisting the keys, you can find the relationship of the bronchi and vessels in any

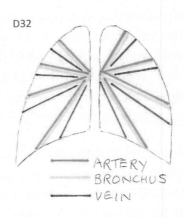

part of the lungs. For example, with the right lung, swing the key up vertically; the pulmonary artery will lie medial to the bronchus and the vein laterally. Swing it down vertically through 180 degrees; the artery will be lateral and the vein medial. Swing it round to the front of the ring; the artery will lie in front of the bronchus with the vein behind. Swing it up through 180 degrees; the artery will lie behind with the vein in front. Swing it round to the back of the ring; the artery will be in front with the vein behind. Swing it down through 180 degrees; the artery will be behind with the vein in front. These manoeuvres can be repeated on the left side to give a mirror image of the positions in the right lung. The exercise could be repeated using a small fan, with the unexpanded blades held horizontally with blue paint on the top and red paint below on each blade. Open the fan into a semi-circle and swivel it forwards and backwards with the same result as with the keys. I noticed that the arteries followed this pattern fairly faithfully, but the relationship of the veins to the bronchi was not so constant. In the upper lobes the bronchi and vessels were crowded together, but in the lower lobes there was more space between them. In the upper lobes the arteries would lie central to the bronchi, with the veins lying peripherally. In the lower lobes the arteries would lie on the outside of the bronchi and the veins on the inner side, with a gradual change from above downwards. D 32.

On 25<sup>th</sup> May 2018, I removed the pleura and lung tissue from the vertebral surface of the lung of a foetal lamb and uncovered the bronchi and vessels. In the upper part the arteries were nearest the surface medially with the bronchi lateral to them. In the middle section the arteries were above the bronchi. In the lowest part the veins were most medial with the bronchi lateral to them. My limited examination of a foetal lung agreed with the arrangement I had seen in the museum. D 33.

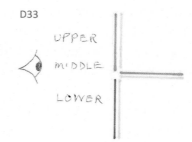

The postnatal lung has a double respiratory circulation: a major pulmonary which drains into the left atrium and feeds the body tissues with oxygen, and a minor bronchial which feeds the bronchi and other tissues of the lung with oxygen and drains into the right atrium. There can be little or no connection between the two systems within the lungs, or the bronchial would lead oxygen into the right atrium and the pulmonary would lead carbon dioxide into the left atrium. The lung tissues are really a special part of the body tissues, concealed within the lungs and fed by oxygen from the pulmonary system which supplies the bronchial arteries. The respiratory capillaries are the most important part of the pulmonary system, which receive oxygen from the air in the adjacent airways. But in the foetus, there is no air in the airways; the pulmonary system cannot feed the body or the lungs with oxygen. The bronchial system continues to feed the lungs with oxygen because the supply now comes from the placenta, but the respiratory capillaries are excluded from this supply because they are part of the pulmonary system. *Now we see why the foetus has a third respiratory system to nourish the respiratory capillaries, which is the unnamed branch from the inferior vena cava, because the other two are excluded from doing so.*

The Liver.

Arterial blood contains food and oxygen. Both are essential for metabolism; one is no good without the other. In the foetus the liver discharges both into the upper part of the inferior vena cava, and some branches off to the lungs, as I have shown earlier. But in the postnate the liver only discharges food, not oxygen; the oxygen is added in the lungs. Between the liver and the lungs therefore, the blood contains only food and carbon-dioxide, and when the blood reaches the respiratory zone of the lungs an equivalent amount of oxygen is exchanged for the carbon-dioxide.

The Block.

It has been difficult for those, who like me have investigated the foetal circulation so deeply obscured. It has often been guesswork; we've all had a go at it. Perhaps the most difficult problem has been the block I have introduced, to separate the venous return of the lower body from the arterial blood in the upper inferior vena cava which feeds the left atrium. I have shown by direct observation and by reasoning that the inferior vena cava does feed the left atrium. I have also shown by some fundamental facts of physiology that the arterial blood in the inferior vena cava cannot be contaminated with the venous return from the lower body. The lower return must reach the right atrium by an alternative route, using the superior vena cava, and the right atrium can have only one vena cava, the superior. Of the few foetal lambs I had examined, one did not have an inferior vena cava leading to the liver, and in the one postnatal lamb there was no inferior vena cava. It appears that in the local breed of sheep the inferior vena cava is an inconstant feature, and in two of the lambs there would have been an alternative route for the lower return.

In the previous edition of this book I had considered the pressure in the umbilical vein and inferior vena cava to be very low; the blood had travelled a long way from the junction to the placenta and back to the heart. I now have other ideas; as the muscular umbilical arteries clasp and pump the umbilical vein, would the pressure within it be raised with each heartbeat?

In the foetus, the diaphragm is higher than in the postnate, with the heart lying high up and occupying most of the space in the narrow chest. Although the liver is an abdominal organ, it also lies high up, probably in a squashed position within the narrow chest wall. The inferior vena cava is intimately connected to the liver and runs behind it. The squashed liver would prevent the venous return from the lower body from flowing to the left atrium in the inferior vena cava, while the raised pressure in the umbilical vein would allow the placental stream to bypass the liver and reach the left atrium. *The Liver is the Block!*

Part Three.

## The Foetal Heart Sounds.

With the long- held view that blood flows through the foramen ovale from the right to left atrium, the valve would be held open, not making a sound until it is closed at birth. But there is a sound as the valve closes with each beat of the heart, as any lady in the later months of pregnancy may confirm with a Doppler foetal heart monitor. The two sounds made by the postnatal heart measure the duration of ventricular systole, with the softer 'lub' heard as the ventricles contract and close the atrioventricular valves, and the harsher 'dup' occurring when the ventricles begin to open and the outlet valves close. The left ventricular sounds are louder than the right sounds, and we need only consider them. The atrioventricular valve is the mitral and the outlet is the aortic. In the foetus there is an extra sound made by the closing of the foramen ovale. It is much softer than the other two and more difficult to hear because atrial muscle is much weaker than ventricular muscle, and when the left atrium contracts in systole the closing valve causes little vibration in the valve and the surrounding blood. But it can be heard nevertheless and occurs just before the other two as the atrium contracts immediately before the onset of ventricular systole. So there will be a triple rhythm; soft lub, louder lub, and harsher dup. Anybody with a Doppler machine should be able to find this rhythm,

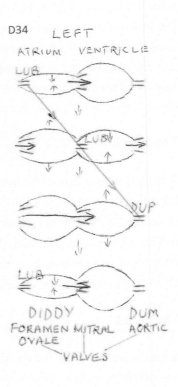

and it is best not to search for the individual sounds close together at a speed of 140 beats per minute; just find the triple gallop rhythm. Move the machine about and you will find the difference between the double rhythm heard in some places and the gallop rhythm heard elsewhere: diddy-dum, diddy-dum, diddy-dum, with a very short diddy. D 34. The left atrium is a posterior structure, as I have said, and the triple rhythm would be more easily heard from the back of the foetus. Also, the flexed position of the foetus would keep the front of the chest away from the probing monitor. The triple rhythm indicates that the left atrium is pumping blood into the left ventricle, but not from the right atrium; it could only come from the inferior vena cava. The right atrium is beating too of course, but it has no inlet valve to contribute to the heart sounds.

With five valves opening and closing, it is quite possible that the four pulmonary valves may contribute to the soft lub of the atrial component of the foetal heart sounds. But without a contribution from the larger foramen ovale, could the four smaller ones contribute to the heart sounds after birth? I looked up my physiology book. There is an 'atrial sound' and I believe it is more likely to be caused by the closing of the pulmonary valves in atrial systole, rather than the explanation given in the book. I will not say more to respect copyright.

Part Four.

## The Birth Changes.

The changes are in two parts: the first during the delivery when the placental circulation is dismantled, and the second when breathing begins.

A bright new light which illuminated the long-hidden secrets of the foetal circulation in April 1965, had been switched on by the death of the little girl who had failed to breathe after her delivery. Why she did not breathe we shall never know, but we will know that the transition from foetus to baby is due to the onset of breathing. The light is never switched on again, and we are kept in the dark during the transition. We can see the external changes: the waking, the breathing and the crying, but the internal changes are shielded from us and have never been seen. But if we have been able to recognise correctly how the foetus differs from the postnate, we will be more able to work out/guess the hidden changes which must occur at birth. As they depend on breathing, they cannot occur in the mother; they take place outside the mother after the delivery. Therefore, the creature which is delivered is a foetus, and the birth of the baby takes place after the delivery when the first deep breath is taken. The little 'girl' who had died in 1965 would also have been a foetus, and it was her foetal features which had shone so brightly on that April day.

It is important to search for any clues which may help us to understand the internal changes which occur during the transition. But first we must consider the situation of the human foetus to be the same as that of the wild animal foetus, without the presence of any professional medical attendants to affect the outcome of the delivery (apart from the mother). Let us go to the beginning and start with the delivery. As it is completed and the foetus leaves the mother, the emptied contracted uterus will squash the placenta and stop the circulation within it and within all the vessels of the cord, and the foetus will be denied a blood supply. This is a clue; the first evidence of a possible change in the internal circulation of the foetus. There will be a double effect, with the stopping of the flow in the umbilical vein to the foetus, and the stopping of the flow in the umbilical arteries to the placenta. There is usually a provisional flow of oxygenated blood into the umbilical vein for the left atrium as the uterus mangles the placenta and wrings out the blood, and this is of benefit for the foetus, but the flow will eventually cease. The effect on the placenta will be more dramatic; there may be pulsation in the umbilical arteries but there can be no flow into the placenta, and the large cardiac output of mixed blood for the placenta will be captured by the foetus and transferred to the lower body. The foetus will therefore gain from the effects on both the umbilical vein and the umbilical arteries and will be well cared for naturally at this time when the placental circulation is dismantled.

Then the breathing begins. But when does it begin, and why does it begin? It is usually accompanied by the arrival of consciousness; we must not forget that. I believe there must be an inhibitory factor which prevents the foetus from waking and breathing in utero, and that after the delivery it is cancelled, and simultaneously another factor, stimulation, causes the foetus to wake and breathe and cry. The shock of entry into the outside world, with the rapid cooling of the naked wet body of the human foetus, like having a cold shower, would seem to be the most obvious external factor. But could the blocked flow to the placenta be an internal factor too?

Let us consider the Venturi at the junction. When the placenta is squashed and the large mixed flow in the umbilical arteries is transferred to the lower body, could there be raised pressure and a reflex in the aorta to the brain which would cause the foetus to wake? And as the large flow of mixed blood passes through the lower body, the arterial portion would be utilised by the tissues and a double flow of venous blood would reach the right atrium. Earlier I have suggested reflex control of respiration by the right atrium in the postnate. Therefore, could the wave of blood reaching the right atrium cause the foetus to breathe? In which case the squashed placenta would stimulate the foetus to wake up and breathe after the delivery when it is safe to do so, and the shock of entry into the outside world come *after* the foetus has woken and breathed, *not before,* and the baby would cry and keep the lungs well aerated immediately after birth. *Foetus delivered, foetus wakes and breathes, baby cries.*

My account of the hidden changes is all guess work, of course, but I have had the benefit of seeing each part of the foetal circulation, which has helped me to work them out. They all happen quickly together at the same time, while I have had to write a description of them one after the other in sequence. They all depend on the expansion of the chest and the descent of the diaphragm when the first deep breath is taken, and all involve the left atrium. *Fundamentally they show that the oxygen for the left atrium which had been delivered from the placenta, comes from the lungs as breathing begins at birth.* Especially important is the strong attachment of the inferior vena cava to the central tendon of the diaphragm which ensures that the circulatory and respiratory changes are perfectly synchronised.

The chest has the shape of a cone with the diaphragm rising steeply from its sides to a highly placed central dome, and with the organs packed closely together contributing to the economy of space in the foetus. When the first deep breath is taken the diaphragm and the organs move down to a wider section of the cone, which becomes even wider with the expansion of the chest wall, and there is a sudden *increase* in the size of the thoracic cage matched by a sudden *decrease* in intra-thoracic pressure. Two fluid components allow the chest and lungs to expand: air entering the respiratory passages from the trachea, and venous blood diverted from the pulmonary trunk to the pulmonary arteries of the lungs. Both are indispensable and quickly meet each other in the respiratory zone of the lung periphery. The air brings oxygen to the lungs, and the blood will carry the oxygen to the left atrium and every part of the body for all its functions. The venous blood diverted from the pulmonary trunk would be the very same blood transferred from the umbilical arteries when the placenta is squashed at the time of delivery. *Now we see the importance of the large circulation to the placenta captured by the foetus; without it the lungs would be unable to expand fully at birth. This diversion of venous blood to the lungs is a major event, with a beneficial massive disruption of the circulation which is the hallmark of the changes, giving the foetus a new life of independence from the mother as it becomes a baby.* The descent of the diaphragm and the expansion of the chest pull down the inferior vena cava and liver to a wider section, remove the block and unite the two parts of the vena cava. At the same time the tissues which separate the upper inferior vena cava from the right atrium are pulled away by the descending diaphragm and the vena cava leads venous blood from the lower body into an enlarged right atrium instead of the departing provisional arterial blood into the left atrium. The foramen ovale is now lying between the right and left atria beating together, and without a flow between them the valve becomes closed, while the arterial supply to the left atrium is replaced by fresh blood coming from the lungs through the pulmonary veins on the other side of the atrium. The great diversion of venous blood from the pulmonary trunk to the lungs suddenly removes the venous blood supply from the ductus arteriosus and the lower body. The ductus, lying beyond the origin of the pulmonary arteries, collapses and closes without a venous blood supply and abolishes the segregated blood supply, while the venous portion of the mixed stream for the lower body also disappears and the lower body is fed only by arterial blood.

It all happens in the twinkling of an eye, invisibly in front of those who are privileged to witness the birth of a baby, at the end of the first deep breath.

It is great theatre: the left atrium occupies centre stage, with dissolution and assembly side by side in each wing as the first deep breath is taken.

On the right, the block on the inferior vena cava is removed, both venae cavae enter the right atrium and all the venous blood is directed into the right ventricle and pulmonary trunk, while the foramen ovale is closed and the left atrium is denied a blood supply.

On the left, the venous blood in the pulmonary trunk is diverted to the lungs and left atrium, with an uninterrupted supply of oxygen for the changing creature, while the supply to the lower body is arterial only. The ductus arteriosus closes and arterial blood is distributed to both parts of the body equally.

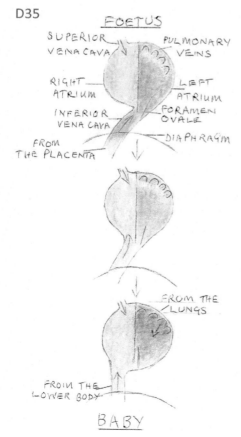

It is likely for the birth changes to be the same in the lamb and the human. But my observations on that little girl who had died in 1965 suggest a difference, which concerns the inferior vena cava carrying arterial blood in the foetus and venous blood in the postnate. Although I was unable to confirm in the anatomy department the close connection between the foramen ovale and the inferior vena cava, I have unearthed some of my early unpublished drawings which do show a close relationship.

The first drawing, made in January 1969, shows the foramen ovale overhanging the vena cava inside the right atrium. The second drawing, probably of the same specimen, again shows this close relationship in the right atrium. In which case the change in the inferior vena cava would occur as I have shown in D 35.

The descending diaphragm pulls the inferior vena cava away from the foramen ovale, closing the valve, and the vena cava leads venous blood into the right atrium, while the arterial blood for the left atrium is replaced by four streams from the other side of the left atrium coming from the lungs.

Perhaps this is what happens in the foetal lamb, but either way the change would be the same.

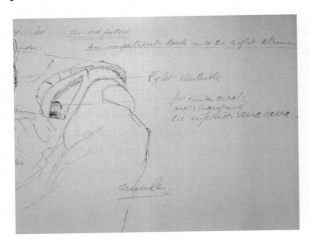 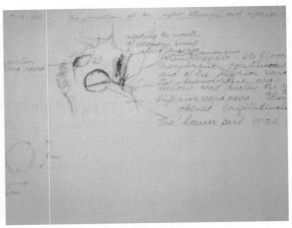

We now see why the postnatal right atrium has two venae cavae, because each foetal atrium has one: the superior for the right atrium and the inferior for the left. At birth, the inferior vena cava switches over to the right atrium, which gains the second one, while the left atrium has no vena cava and its blood supply is replaced by fresh blood coming through the four pulmonary veins from the lungs.

The postnatal respiratory rate is about twelve breaths per minute, five seconds for each breath, I say two for inspiration and three for expiration. I am not sure how long the first deep breath would last, but it would probably be only for a second or two. At the beginning of the first deep breath the creature would be a foetus, and at the end, only a second or two later it would be a baby. That is how long all those changes I have described would take, perfectly synchronised by the strong attachment of the inferior vena cava to the central tendon of the diaphragm.

When the first deep *expiration* is taken the organs do not return to their foetal position but take up a new fixed lower position from where all future respiratory excursions will be made. There are other changes too: the heart becomes more vertical and the heart rate is decreased, with loss of the atrial sound and the gallop rhythm. The panicky crying stops as the baby is comforted on the breast, and quiet breathing begins. Very soon there will be a wet or soiled nappy as the three functions of the placenta are taken over by the lungs, the kidneys and the alimentary tract.

D 36 is the first of five diagrams illustrating the birth changes: the first three in the foetus and the last two in the baby. The first shows a modified plan of the circulation in the foetus before any of the birth changes have occurred. The placental supply of mixed blood is much larger than that for the lower body and the blood meeting the placental interface is venous, not mixed. Vide supra, The Circulation for the Placenta and the Plan of the Circulation.

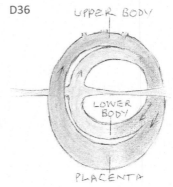

D 37 shows the foetus being delivered and the squashed placenta closing the umbilical vessels.

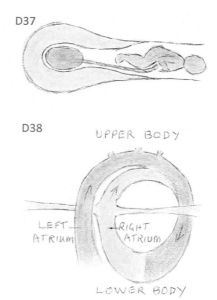

D 38 shows what I believe happens to the circulation when the foetus is delivered. The placenta is squashed, preventing flow down the umbilical arteries, and the large flow of mixed blood to the placenta is transferred to the lower body where it is changed to venous and reaches the right atrium. The squashed placenta squeezes blood into the umbilical vein and the left atrium continues to receive oxygenated arterial blood. Both atria therefore benefit at the time of the delivery, and the placental circulation is dismantled naturally before the midwife or obstetrician can do so. At the same time, the brain is informed that the foetus has been delivered and stimulates the foetus to wake, and the venous flow to the right atrium stimulates the foetus to breathe, when it will rapidly change the circulation into that of the baby.

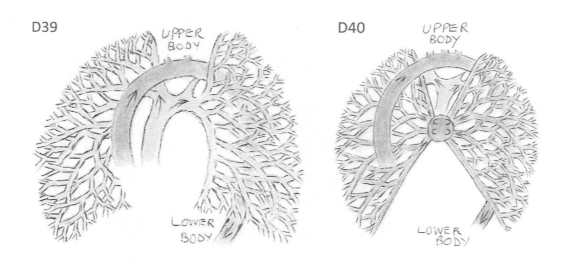

D 39 shows how the first deep breath diverts the venous blood from the pulmonary trunk to the periphery of the lungs and changes the circulation into that of the baby. *This is when the baby is born, at the end of the first deep breath.* The ductus arteriosus collapses and closes without a venous blood supply, and the lower body is fed with arterial blood.

D 40. In the next heartbeat or two, the blood has been oxygenated and has reached the left atrium, from where it will spread to all parts of the baby and return as venous to the right atrium, right ventricle and pulmonary trunk.

During the transition from foetus to baby, the blood supply for the lower body changes from mixed to arterial, but the left atrium and upper body are well supplied with arterial blood throughout.

In the foetus, D 41, the arterial supply for the left atrium comes from the placenta and the inferior vena cava, but in the baby, D 42, the inferior vena cava feeds the right atrium with venous blood, and the arterial supply for the left atrium comes from the lungs.

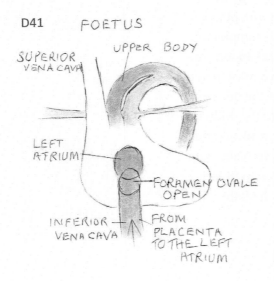

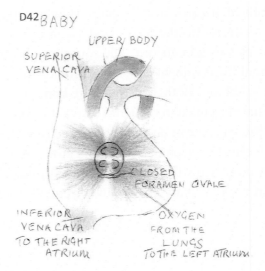

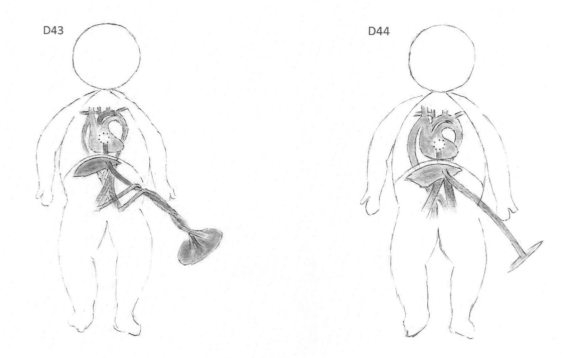

D 43 shows the foetus before labour has begun. D 44 when the foetus is delivered.

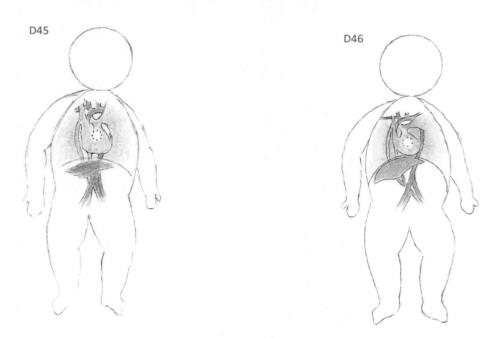

D 45 when the foetus wakes up and breathes. D 46 after the first deep breath when the baby cries.

*Foetus delivered, foetus wakes and breathes, baby cries.*

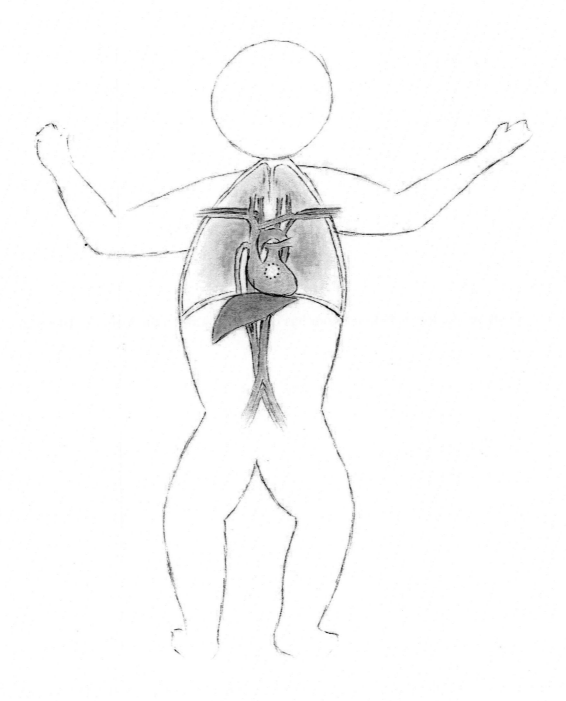

The shock of entering the outside world does not make the
baby cry. It is the shock of leaving the mother.
Birth is an intrinsic, intimate process between the mother, the foetus and the baby.

Printed in the United States
by Baker & Taylor Publisher Services